© **2023 KIKI BROWN.** All rights reserved. No part of this ebook may be reproduced, distributed, or transmitted in any form or by any means, including photocopying, recording, or other electronic or mechanical methods, without the prior written permission of the author/publisher, except in the case of brief quotations embodied in critical reviews and certain other noncommercial uses permitted by copyright law

Table of Contents

INTRODUCTION

Menopause officially begins when you've gone 12 consecutive months without menstruating. Symptoms like night sweats are common right before, during, and after menopause. Treatment can help manage them. Menopause occurs from hormone changes as the body nears the end of its reproductive years. After menopause, you will have no more periods. In the United States, menopause happens on average at age 52 years but it may occur earlier or later. Menopause can cause symptoms such as hot flashes and weight changes. Treatment can help manage these symptoms.

Stages of menopause

Menopause symptoms usually start about 4 years before the final period. Symptoms can continue for several years, depending on the person. Perimenopause is when your hormones begin to change before menopause. It often begins after the mid-40sTrusted Source and can last anywhere from a few months to several years. Early menopause is when menopause occurs at ages 40–45 years. About 5% of females experience early menopause. Premature menopause or primary ovarian insufficiency is when menopause begins before age 40 years.

What are the symptoms of menopause?

Everyone's experience of menopause is unique. Some people experience severe and wide-ranging symptoms, while others may barely notice the change. Apart from the presence or absence of menstruation, the symptoms of perimenopause, menopause, and postmenopause are similar. The most common early symptoms of perimenopause are:

less frequent menstruation

heavier or lighter periods than usual

vasomotor symptoms, including hot flashes, night sweats, and flushing

Hot flashes last on average 5.2 yearsTrusted Source, starting around a year before menopause. They usually lessen after menopause but can persist for up to 20 years. They affect 70–80% of people experiencing menopause. Other common symptoms of menopause include:

insomnia

vaginal dryness

weight gain

depression

anxiety

difficulty concentrating

memory problems

reduced libido, or sex drive

dry skin, mouth, and eyes

increased urination

sore or tender breasts

headaches

racing heart

urinary tract infections (UTIs)

reduced muscle mass

painful or stiff joints

reduced bone mass

less full breasts

hair thinning or loss

increased hair growth on other areas of the body, such as the face, neck, chest, and upper back

Complications

Around the same time that menopause happens, the chances of various other health-related issues increase. It can be hard to distinguish the complications of menopause and those related to aging. Some complications or health changes you may experience around this time include:

vulvovaginal atrophy

dyspareunia, or painful intercourse

osteoporosis, or weaker bones with reduced mass and strength

mood or sudden emotional changes

urinary incontinence

heart or blood vessel disease

weight gain and change in body composition

Why does menopause occur?

Menopause is a natural process that results from changing levelsTrusted Source of estrogen, progesterone, and other hormones as you age. These changes are linked to a loss of active ovarian follicles. These structures produce and release eggs from the ovary wall and allow menstruation and fertility. In some cases, menopause occurs early from surgery, radiation therapy, chemotherapy, a pelvic injury, or other factors affecting the reproductive organs. This is called induced menopause.

Anyone assigned female at birth will likely experience menopause at some time. Gender transition surgery or hormone treatment may bring on menopause during or after treatment. Changes in the levels of certain hormones can induce symptoms of menopause regardless of a person's gender or sex assigned at birth.

How is menopause diagnosed?

Most people know they are approaching or starting menopause when they begin having symptoms such as hot flashes or when they have not had a period for 12 months. Not everyone needs to seek medical advice during menopause. If you do, however, a doctor may use a blood test to confirm if menopause is likely. These tests can include the following:

The PicoAMH Elisa diagnostic test can help determineTrusted Source whether menopause has begun.

Other blood tests can measure levels of FSH and estradiol, a form of estrogen. Blood levels that are consistently 30 mIU/mL or higher, combined with a lack of menstruation for 1 year, can usually confirm menopause.

Saliva tests and over-the-counter (OTC) urine tests are also available, but they can be expensive and are not always reliable.

Depending on your symptoms and health history, a doctor may also order additional blood tests to help rule out other underlying conditions that may causing your symptoms. These tests can include:

thyroid function tests

blood lipid profile

liver function tests

kidney function tests

testosterone, progesterone, prolactin, estradiol, and chorionic gonadotropin (hCG) tests

It's worth seeking medical help if menopause symptoms are affecting your daily life, you have other symptoms not related to menopause, or you're experiencing menopause symptoms and are younger than age 45 years.

Treatments

Treatment for menopause symptoms include:

hormonal treatments to help manage hot flashes and other symptoms

lubricants for vaginal dryness

supplements and medications to help prevent osteoporosis

If you experience discomfort as menopause approaches, talk with a doctor. They can guide you through the process and provide treatments that help manage your symptoms.

Home remedies and lifestyle strategies

Some lifestyle strategies and home or alternative treatments can also help manage some menopause symptoms.

Keep cool and stay comfortable

Dress in loose, layered clothing that you can remove or put on easily to help manage hot flashes.

Keep your bedroom cool and avoid heavy blankets to reduce night sweats.

Carry a portable fan to help cool you down when you feel flushed.

Exercise

Current guidelinesTrusted Source recommend getting at least 150 minutes of moderate exercise and two sessions of resistance training per week.

Exercise can help strengthen your body, boost overall well-being, and manage weight.

Communicate your needs and get support

Mental health concerns, such as depression, anxiety, sadness, and isolation, can occur during menopause.

You can try talking with family or friends, joining a local support group, or seeking counseling to help you manage the changes that are occurring.

A 2023 research review suggests dietary choices during menopause can help manage depression, weight, skin changes, and even vasomotor symptoms. Getting a variety of essential nutrients through a varied, balanced diet can boost your overall well-being during menopause.

Supplements

Herbs and supplements may help Dietary choices
manage some effects of menopause. For instance, calcium, vitamin D, and magnesium may help reduce the risk of osteoporosis. Ask a doctor for advice on supplements for your individual needs. A doctor can also make sure a supplement will not interact with any medications you may be taking.

Manage stress

Techniques for managing stress include relaxation and breathing exercises, such as:

yoga

box breathing

meditation

How can menopause affect your mental health?

Take care of your skin

Apply moisturizers daily to reduce skin dryness. Try to avoid excessive sun exposure and harsh cosmetics and cleansing products, too. They may dry out your skin. How does your skin change during menopause and what can you do about it?

Manage sleeping issues

Getting enough sleep is essential for overall health and well-being.Talk with your doctor if you regularly have trouble sleeping. They can help you manage it and get a better night's rest.

Avoid smoking and limit alcohol use

If you smoke, it might be a good time to quit smoking and take measures to avoid exposure to secondhand smoke to protect your overall health. A high alcohol intake may make you feel worse as well. Limiting alcohol consumption to no more than one drink per dayTrusted Source can help prevent a range of health issues.

Other remedies

Some people use alternative remedies to increase estrogen levels, but there's not enough evidence to prove they are safe or effective. These alternative remedies include:

soy isoflavones

vitamins, such as vitamin E

melatonin

flaxseed

Some people use black cohosh to improve symptoms such as hot flashes and night sweats. However, there is little evidenceTrusted Source to support these claims. More research is needed. Some researchTrusted Source suggests omega-3 fatty acids may help improve night sweats but not hot flashes or other symptoms.

WHAT IS MENOPAUSE?

Anything that damages your ovaries or stops estrogen production can cause early menopause. This includes chemotherapy for cancer or an oophorectomy (removal of the ovaries).In these cases, your doctor will help prepare you for early menopause. But your body can also start menopause early even if your ovaries are still inside you.

Language matters

Sex and gender exist on spectrums. We use "women" in this article to refer to sex assigned at birth.

What are the symptoms of early menopause?

Early menopause can begin as soon as you start having irregular periods or periods that are noticeably longer or shorter than your typical cycle. Other symptoms of early menopause include:

heavy bleeding

spotting

periods that last longer than a week

a longer amount of time inbetween periods

In these cases, contact your doctor to check for any other issues that might be causing these symptoms. Other common symptoms of menopause include:

mood swings

changes in sexual feelings or desire

vaginal dryness

trouble sleeping

hot flashes

night sweats

loss of bladder control

What causes early menopause?

There are several known causes of early menopause, but sometimes the cause cannot be determined.

Genetics

If there's no obvious medical reason for early menopause, the cause is likely genetic. Your age at menopause onset is likely inherited. Knowing when your parent started menopause can provide clues about when you'll start your own. If your parent started menopause early, you're more likely than average to do the same. However, genes tell only half the story.

Lifestyle factors

Some lifestyle factors may have an impact on when you begin menopause. Smoking affects estrogen and can contribute to early menopause. Some researchTrusted Source suggests that long-term or regular smokers are likely to experience menopause sooner. Women who smoke may start menopause 1 to 2 years earlier than women who don't smoke. Body mass index (BMI) can also factor into early menopause. Estrogen is stored in fat tissue. Women who are very thin have fewer estrogen stores, which can be depleted sooner. Some research also suggests that a vegetarian diet, lack of exercise, and lack of sun exposure throughout your life can all cause an early onset of menopause.

Chromosome issues

Some chromosomal issues can lead to early menopause. For example, Turner syndrome (also called monosomy X and gonadal dysgenesis) involves being born with an incomplete chromosome. Women with Turner syndrome have ovaries that don't function as expected. This often causes them to enter menopause prematurely. Other chromosomal issues can cause early menopause, too. This includes pure gonadal dysgenesis, a variation on Turner syndrome.

In this condition, the ovaries don't function. Instead, periods and secondary sex characteristics must be brought about by hormone replacement therapy, usually during adolescence. Women with Fragile X syndrome, or who are genetic carriers of the disease, may also have early menopause. This syndrome is passed down in families. You can discuss genetic testing options with your doctor if you have premature menopause or if you have family members who had premature menopause.

Autoimmune diseases

Premature menopause can be a symptom of an autoimmune disease, such as thyroid disease or rheumatoid arthritis. In autoimmune diseases, the immune system mistakes a part of the body for an invader and attacks it. Inflammation caused by some of these diseases can affect the ovaries. Menopause begins when the ovaries stop working.

Epilepsy

Epilepsy is a seizure disorder that stems from the brain. Someone with epilepsy is more likely to experience primary ovarian insufficiency, which leads to menopause. Changing hormone levels due to menopause can affect seizures in people with epilepsy. An older study from 2001Trusted Source found that in a group of women with epilepsy, about 14 percent of those studied had premature menopause, as opposed to 1 percent of the general population.

How is early menopause diagnosed?

The time leading into menopause is called perimenopause. During this time, you may have irregular periods and other symptoms that come and go. You're generally considered to be in menopause if you go 12 months without menstrual bleeding, and you don't have another medical condition to explain your symptoms. This may be an indicator of early menopause.

Testing for early menopause

Tests aren't usually needed to diagnose menopause. Most people can self-diagnose menopause based on their symptoms. But if you think you're experiencing early menopause, you may want to contact your doctor to be sure. Your doctor can order hormone tests to help determine whether your symptoms are due to perimenopause or another condition. These are the most common hormones to check: Anti-Müllerian hormone (AMH). The PicoAMH Elisa testTrusted Source uses this hormone to help determine whether you're approaching menopause or have already reached your last menstrual cycle.

Estrogen. Your doctor may check your levels of estrogen, also called estradiol. In menopause, estrogen levels decrease.

Follicle-stimulating hormone (FSH). If your FSH levels are consistently above 30 milli-international units per milliliter (mIU/mL), and you haven't menstruated for a year, it's likely that you've reached menopause. However, a single elevated FSH test can't confirm menopause on its own.

Thyroid-stimulating hormone (TSH). Your doctor may check your levels of TSH to confirm diagnosis. If you have an underactive thyroid (hypothyroidism), you'll have TSH levels that are too high. Symptoms of the condition are similar to the symptoms of menopause.

The North American Menopause Society (NAMS) reports that hormone tests are sometimes unhelpful because hormone levels still change and fluctuate during perimenopause.

Even so, if you're concerned about signs of menopause, NAMS suggests requesting a full checkup with your doctor.

How is early menopause treated or managed?
Early menopause generally doesn't require treatment. However, there are treatment options available to help manage the symptoms of menopause or conditions related to it. They can help you deal with changes in your body or lifestyle more easily. Premature menopause is often treated because it occurs at such an early age. This helps support your body with the hormones it would typically make until you reach the age of natural menopause.

The most common treatment includes hormone replacement therapy (HRT). Systemic hormone therapy can prevent many common menopausal symptoms. Or you may take vaginal hormone products, usually in low doses, to help with vaginal symptoms. HRT does have risks though. It can increase your chances of:

heart disease

stroke

breast cancer

Talk with your doctor about the risks and benefits of your individual care before starting HRT. Lower doses of hormones may decrease your risk of experiencing these conditions.

Lifestyle and home remedies

Although you can't prevent menopause from happening, you can take action to help your symptoms. Eating a healthy diet and exercising regularly can help manage menopause symptoms. If you smoke, consider quitting to manage your symptoms as well. There is mixed evidence on using natural products to manage menopause symptoms. Some people prefer vitamins and herbal supplements over conventional medication. Check with your doctor about which treatment is right for you.

Can early menopause be reversed?

For now, available treatment can help delay or reduce the symptoms of menopause, but there is no sure way to reverse early menopause. However, researchers are investigating new ways to help people in menopause have children. In 2016, scientists in Greece announced a new treatment that enabled them to restore menstruation and retrieve eggs from a small group of women who were in perimenopause. This treatment made headlines as a way to "reverse" menopause, but little is known about how well it works.

The scientists reported treating more than 30 women, ages 46 to 49, by injecting platelet-rich plasma (PRP) into their ovaries. PRP is sometimes used to promote tissue healing, but the treatment hasn't been proven to be effective for any purpose. The scientists claimed the treatment worked for two-thirds of the women treated. However, the research has been criticized for its small size and lack of control groups. Though the research might have potential for the future, it's not a realistic treatment option right now.

Can early menopause contribute to other conditions?

Infertility is often a big concern when you start menopause 10 or more years early. Yet, there are other health concerns. A steady stream of estrogen to your tissues has many uses. Estrogen increases "good" HDL cholesterol and decreases "bad" LDL cholesterol. It also relaxes blood vessels and prevents bones from thinning. Losing estrogen earlier than typical can increase your risk of:

heart disease

osteoporosis

depression

dementia

premature death

If you have concerns about these symptoms, speak with your doctor. Because of these risks, people who enter menopause early are often prescribed HRT.

Can early menopause protect you from other conditions?

Starting menopause early can actually protect you from other diseases. These include estrogen-sensitive cancers such as breast cancer. People who enter menopause late (after age 55) are at greater risk of breast cancer than those who enter the transition earlier. This is because their breast tissue is exposed to estrogen for a longer time.

Easing the transition to menopause

A genetic test may one day determine a person's likelihood of early menopause. For now, though, only time will tell when you'll start your transition. Contact your doctor for regular checkups, and try to be proactive about your reproductive health. Doing so can help your doctor ease the symptoms or decrease your risk factors for early menopause.Seeing a therapist can also help you cope with any pain or anxiety you may feel during menopause.

Fertility and your options

If you're interested in having children, you still have a few options for growing your family. These include:

adoption

receiving an egg donation

having a surrogate carry your child

A fertility specialist may also suggest procedures that can help you have children. Talk with your doctor about the options available to you for becoming a parent. Their risks and successes can be affected by many factors, including your age and overall health.

Understanding How Your Skin Changes During Menopause

If you've shopped for skin care online or in a store recently, you know there are tons of "anti-aging" products available. While a serum or cream can only do so much, there's no denying that skin changes with age. Skin ages for several reasons. Ultraviolet (UV) ray exposure over time breaks down elastin, which can make skin lose its elasticity. Fat under the skin can shrink too, leading to a loss of plumpness or sagging. But another factor in skin changes is menopause.

What skin changes occur during menopause?

Menopause doesn't happen overnight. It's officially defined as going 1 year without a period. While the timing is unique from person to person, it occurs on average at age 51. This hormonal change causes many side effects, including:

hot flashes

fatigue

vaginal dryness or pain

Skin changes during menopause are very common. You may notice that before and during this time, your skin feels dry and thin, or you may begin to see more wrinkles. Some people may experience acne during menopause as a result of hormonal fluctuations.

What are common skin conditions with menopause?

When the production of hormones estrogen and progesterone rapidly drop off with menopause, most people see it in their skin. The skin may become dry or less plump. Hot flashes can also cause redness, and changing hormone levels may cause acne. According to the American Academy of Dermatology, collagen drops 30% in the first 5 years of menopause, then approximately another 2% each year for the next 20 or so years.

Why does skin change during menopause?

It may be frustrating to notice skin changes during menopause, but it's very typical Collagen is what gives skin plumpness and structure. The rapid loss of collagen can lead to fine lines and wrinkles or cause sagging in the cheeks. Dry skin and acne are also common. Estrogen helps skin produce oil and hold onto water, so extremely dry skin during menopause is common thanks to a drop in this hormone. Some people will also notice acne as estrogen levels fall and androgen levels remain stable (androgens are male sex hormones, like testosterone), increasing sebum production and causing pores to become blocked.

Can you prevent skin changes during menopause?

Menopause is inevitable and healthy for a person with a uterus, but that doesn't mean they'll love the side effects, including skin changes. You may not be able to prevent menopause from taking a toll on your skin, but you can certainly take steps at home to make your skin look its best.

Because one of the main factors in skin aging is sun exposure, it's essential to wear SPF daily — even when it's cloudy. To help keep hormonal acne at bay, use a cleanser with salicylic acid. This can penetrate pores and dissolve oil. Hydration is also important for menopausal skin. It's likely that your face and body will feel drier than usual, and using a moisturizer with hyaluronic acid may help draw moisture into the skin It's best to use moisturizers with hyaluronic acid on damp skin so the ingredient can bond with water. A moisturizer with ceramides can help moisture from escaping, and topping a moisturizer with a facial oil adds even more hydration.

In addition to skin care products, it's always helpful to eat hydrating foods, drink plenty of water, and try to get quality sleep.

There also appears to be a relation between skin appearance postmenopause and race. In a 2021 studyTrusted Source, Black women had fewer wrinkle scores compared with white women 4 years postmenopause.

What are the treatments for skin changes during menopause?

If the skin changes from menopause are really bothering you and are paired with other symptoms, like vaginal dryness, your doctor may suggest hormone replacement therapy (HRT). In some cases, if HRT doesn't seem right, they may recommend an herbal alternative to HRT, like valerian root, or dietary changes that may help balance hormones.

BOTOX treatments may also help minimize the appearance of wrinkles.

If you're noticing an increase in facial hair as a result of menopause, laser hair removal may be a good option.

What can you do at home for skin changes during menopause?

Skin care gets more and more advanced all the time, with new formulas and brands popping up. The simplest home remedy for menopausal skin is a good moisturizer. Incorporating pro-aging ingredients, like retinol, vitamin C, glycolic and lactic acids, and of course, SPF will also help. Also make sure to stay hydrated, get enough sleep, and limit your consumption of alcohol, caffeine, and processed or greasy foods.

What's the outlook for people who have skin changes during menopause?

Most people will experience side effects of menopause, including skin changes like dryness. Because of the rapid drop in estrogen, changes may be most noticeable during the onset of menopause when collagen production abruptly drops off. After a few years, skin changes as a result of menopause will feel more gradual.

PREMENOPAUSE, PERIMENOPAUSE, AND MENOPAUSE

Perimenopause and menopause are both transitional phases that indicate an end to your reproductive years. Premenopause, on the other hand, is when there are no symptoms of either. Although this life stage is well known, there are actually different stages within menopause that are important to recognize and understand. Menopause itself officially occurs when you stop menstruating. Perimenopause, on the other hand, means "around menopause." It's also known as the menopause transitional phase and is called such because it happens before menopause. Although they're both part of the same overall life transition, menopause and

Premenopause vs. perimenopause

Premenopause and perimenopause are sometimes used interchangeably, but technically they have different meanings. Premenopause is when you have no symptoms

of perimenopause or menopause. You still have periods —
whether they're regular or irregular — and are considered
to be in your reproductive years. Some hormonal changes
may be occurring, but there are no noticeable changes in
your body. On the other hand, during perimenopause,
you'll start to experience symptoms of menopause. They
may include:

changes in your period cycle

hot flashes

sleep disturbances

mood swings

When perimenopause occurs

Perimenopause occurs well before you officially hit
menopause. In fact, according to the Cleveland Clinic,
hormonal changes are seen 8 to 10 years ahead of
menopause. This happens during your 30s or 40s even
before the onset of perimenopause. Perimenopause is
marked by a drop in estrogen, the main female hormone
produced by the ovaries. The estrogen levels can also go up
and down more sporadically than they do in a typical 28-

day cycle. This can cause irregular periods and other symptoms.

During the final stages of perimenopause, your body will produce less and less estrogen. Despite the sharp drop in estrogen, it's still possible to get pregnant. Perimenopause can last for as little as a few months and as long as 4 years. Menopause officially kicks in when the ovaries produce so little estrogen that eggs are no longer released. This also causes your period to stop. Your doctor will diagnose menopause once you haven't had a period for a full year. You may enter menopause earlier than normal if you:

have a family history of early menopause

are a smoker

have had a hysterectomy or oophorectomy

have undergone cancer treatments

Symptoms of perimenopause and menopause

When it comes to menopause, most people think about the symptoms more than anything else. These can include those infamous hot flashes, but there are many other changes you might experience during this transition.

Perimenopause symptoms

Symptoms of perimenopause may include:

irregular periods

periods that are heavier or lighter than normal

worse premenstrual syndrome (PMS) before periods

breast tenderness

weight gain

hair changes

heart palpitations

headaches

loss of sex drive

concentration difficulties

forgetfulness

muscle aches

urinary tract infections (UTIs)

fertility issues in women who are trying to conceive

Menopause symptoms

As estrogen levels drop, you might start experiencing symptoms of menopause. Some of these can occur while you're still at the perimenopause stage.

night sweats

hot flashes

depression

anxiety or irritability

mood swings

insomnia

fatigue

dry skin

vaginal dryness

frequent urination

Cholesterol

Perimenopause and menopause can also increase cholesterol levels. This is one reason why women in postmenopause are at an even higher risk for heart disease. Continue to have your cholesterol levels measured at least once a year.

When to call a doctor

You don't necessarily have to call your doctor to obtain a perimenopause or menopause diagnosis, but there are instances when you should definitely see your OB-GYN. Call right away if you experience:

spotting after your period

blood clots during your period

bleeding after sex

periods that are much longer or much shorter than normal

Some possible explanations are hormonal imbalances or fibroids, both of which are treatable. However, you also want to rule out the possibility of cancer. You should also call your doctor if the symptoms of either perimenopause or menopause become severe enough to interfere with your daily life.

Treatments for perimenopause and menopause

There are both prescription and over-the-counter (OTC) treatments available for perimenopause and menopause.

Estrogen

Estrogen (hormone) therapy works by normalizing estrogen levels so sudden hormonal spikes and drops don't cause uncomfortable symptoms. Some forms of estrogen may even help reduce the risk of osteoporosis. Estrogen is available over the counter or by prescription. Of note, the Food and Drug Administration (FDA) may not regulate some of the OTC options. Estrogen is usually combined with progestin and comes in many forms, including:

oral pills

creams

gels

skin patches

Shop for over-the-counter estrogen therapy.

Other medications

Other menopause medications are more targeted. For example:

Prescription vaginal creams can alleviate dryness as well as pain from intercourse.

Antidepressants can help with mood swings.

The seizure medication gabapentin (Neurontin) can be an option for hot flashes.

Home remedies for perimenopause and menopause

There are also methods you can use to alleviate your symptoms at home. Regular exercise can help improve your mood, weight gain issues, and even (ironically) your hot flashes. Plan to include some form of physical activity in your daily routine. Just don't work out before bedtime, as this can increase insomnia. Getting enough rest can seem impossible if you're dealing with insomnia. Try doing a relaxing activity right before bed, such as gentle yoga or a warm bath. Avoid daytime naps, as this can interfere with your ability to sleep at night. Here are a few other methods you can try to relieve symptoms:

Pay attention to your diet and avoid large meals.

Quit smoking, if you smoke.

Only drink alcohol in moderation.

Limit caffeine to small quantities and only have it in the morning.

Perimenopause and menopause are both transitional phases that indicate an end to your reproductive years. There are certainly adjustments to be made, but remember that not all aspects are negative.

With all of the available treatments, you can get through these stages more comfortably with a bit more freedom, too. During perimenopause, your levels of the hormones estrogen and progesterone fluctuate. These changes can affect your cycle, leading to irregular or missed periods, and more.

Understanding perimenopause

Menopause refers to the end of your menstrual cycle. Once you've gone 12 months without a period, you've reached menopause. The average woman goes through menopause at 51 years old. The time period before menopause is called perimenopause. Perimenopause symptoms occur for 4 years, on average. However, perimenopause can last anywhere from a few months to 10 years. During this time, the hormones estrogen and progesterone are in flux. Your levels will fluctuate from month to month. These shifts can be erratic, affecting ovulation and the rest of your cycle. You may notice anything from irregular or missed periods to different bleeding patterns. Other symptoms of perimenopause include:

hot flashes

night sweats

sleep troubles

memory issues

difficulty urinating

vaginal dryness

changes in sexual desire or satisfaction

Here's what you can expect from perimenopause and what you can do.

1. Spotting between periods

If you notice some blood on your underwear between periods that doesn't require the use of a pad or tampon, it's likely spotting. Spotting is usually the result of your body's changing hormones and the buildup of your endometrium, or uterine lining. Many women spot before their period starts or as it ends. Mid-cycle spotting around ovulation is also common. If you're regularly spotting every 2 weeks, it may be a sign of a hormonal imbalance. You may want to speak with your healthcare provider.

What you can do

Consider keeping a journal to track your periods. Include information such as:

when they start

how long they last

how heavy they are

whether you have any in-between spotting

You can also log this information in an app, like Eve. Worried about leaks and stains? Consider wearing panty liners. Disposable panty liners are available at most drugstores. They come in a variety of lengths and materials. You can even buy reusable liners that are made of fabric and can be washed over and over again.

2. Abnormally heavy bleeding

When your estrogen levels are high in comparison to your progesterone levels, your uterine lining builds. This results in heavier bleeding during your period as your lining sheds. A skipped period can also cause the lining to build up, leading to heavy bleeding. Bleeding is considered heavy if it:

soaks through one tampon or pad an hour for several hours

requires double protection — such as a tampon and pad — to control menstrual flow

causes you to interrupt your sleep to change your pad or tampon

lasts longer than 7 days

When bleeding is heavy, it may last longer, disrupting your everyday life. You may find it uncomfortable to exercise or carry on with your normal tasks. Heavy bleeding can also cause fatigue and increase your risk for other health concerns, such as anemia.

What you can do

As you may know, taking ibuprofen (Advil, Midol, Motrin) during your period can help with menstrual cramps. If you take it when you're bleeding heavily, it may also reduce your flow. Try taking 200 milligrams (mg) every 4 to 6 hours during the day. If cramps and pain continue, talk to your healthcare provider about hormonal approaches to treatment. Some women have a medical or family history that discourages the use of hormones in the perimenopausal period.

3. Brown or dark blood

The colors you see in your menstrual flow can range from bright red to dark brown, especially toward the end of your period. Brown or dark blood is a sign of old blood exiting the body. Women in perimenopause may also see brown spotting or discharge at other times throughout the month. You may also notice changes in discharge texture. Your discharge may be thin and watery, or it may be clumpy and thick.

What you can do

If you're concerned about your menstrual flow, you may want to schedule an appointment to see your doctor. The variation in color is usually due to the amount of time it takes for the blood and tissue to cycle out of the body, but it can sometimes be a sign of another underlying condition. there's a foul odor to the vaginal discharge, it may be a sign of infection. See your healthcare provider.

4. Shorter cycles

When your estrogen levels are low, your uterine lining is thinner. Bleeding, as a result, may be lighter and last fewer days. Short cycles are more common in the earlier stages of perimenopause. For example, you may have a period that's 2 or 3 days shorter than normal. Your whole cycle may also last 2 or 3 weeks instead of 4. It isn't uncommon to feel like your period just ended when the next one comes.

What you can do

If you're worried about short, unpredictable cycles, consider leakage protection such as liners, pads, or period underwear like Thinx. Pass on tampons and menstrual cups unless you have a menstrual flow. Insertion can be difficult or uncomfortable without this lubrication. You're also more likely to forget to change your tampon or cup, increasing your risk for complications.

5. Longer cycles

In the later stages of perimenopause, your cycles may become much longer and farther apart. Longer cycles are defined as those longer than 38 daysTrusted Source. They're related to anovulatory cycles, or cycles in which you don't ovulate. A 2008 studyTrusted Source suggests that women who experience anovulatory cycles may have lighter bleeding than women who experience ovulatory cycles.

What you can do

If you're dealing with longer cycles, it may be time to invest in a good menstrual cup or a cycle set of blood-wicking underwear. You can also use pads or tampons to help you avoid leakage.

6. Missed cycles

Your fluctuating hormones may also be to blame for a missed cycle. In fact, your cycles may become so far apart that you can't recall the last time you bled. After you've missed 12 consecutive cycles, you've reached menopause. If your cycles are still making an appearance — however delayed — ovulation is still occurring. This means you can still have a period, and you can still get pregnant.Anovulatory cycles can also create delayed or missed periods.

What you can do

Missed cycles every so often usually aren't cause for concern. If you've missed a few consecutive cycles, you may want to take a pregnancy test to determine whether your symptoms are tied to perimenopause.Other early symptoms of pregnancy include:

nausea

breast tenderness

frequent urination

sensitivity to smells

heartburn

You can also make an appointment with your doctor instead of taking a home test. Your doctor can run tests to determine whether you're experiencing symptoms of perimenopause, menopause, or pregnancy. If you aren't pregnant and don't want to conceive, use birth control every time you have sex. Fertility doesn't end until you've completely reached menopause. Use condoms and other barrier methods to prevent sexually transmitted infections (STIs).

7. Overall irregularity

Between long cycles, short cycles, spotting, and heavy bleeding, your cycles during perimenopause may be generally irregular. They may not settle into any discernible pattern, especially as you get closer to menopause. This can be unsettling and frustrating.

What you can do

Try your best to remember that the changes you're experiencing are part of a bigger transition. Just as it began, the process will eventually end when you stop ovulating and reach menopause. In the meantime:

Consider wearing black underwear or investing in period underwear to reduce your risk of stained clothing.

Consider wearing disposable or reusable panty liners to protect from irregular leaks, spotting, and otherwise unexpected bleeding.

Track your periods as best you can via a calendar or an app.

Take notes about abnormal bleeding, pain, discomfort, or other symptoms you're experiencing.

When to see your doctor
In some cases, irregular bleeding may be a sign of another underlying condition. See your doctor if you're also experiencing these symptoms:

extremely heavy bleeding that requires you to change your pad or tampon every hour or two

bleeding that lasts longer than 7 days

bleeding — not spotting — that happens more frequently than every 3 weeks

At your appointment, your doctor will ask about your medical history and about any symptoms you've had. From there, they may give you a pelvic exam and order tests (such as a blood test, a biopsy, or an ultrasound) to rule out more serious issues.

11 NATURAL REMEDIES FOR MENOPAUSE RELIEF

Eating a nutritious diet rich in fruits, vegetables, and protein, among other nutrients, and getting regular physical activity may provide relief from menopause symptoms. During this time, at least two-thirds of menopausal people experience symptoms of menopause. These include hot flashes, night sweats, mood changes, irritability, and tiredness.

In addition, menopausal people are at higher risk of several diseases, including osteoporosis, obesity, heart disease, and diabetes (2). Many people turn to natural supplements and remedies for relief. Here's a list of 11 natural ways to reduce the symptoms of menopause.

1. Eat foods rich in calcium and vitamin D

Hormonal changes during menopause can cause bones to weaken, increasing the risk of osteoporosis. Calcium and vitamin D are linked to good bone health, so it's important to get enough of these nutrients in your diet.bAdequate vitamin D intake during postmenopause is also associated with a lower risk of hip fractures from weak bones (4). Many foods are calcium-rich, including dairy products like yogurt, milk, and cheese.

Green, leafy vegetables such as kale, collard greens, and spinach have lots of calcium too. It's also plentiful in tofu, beans, sardines, and other foods. Additionally, calcium-fortified foods are also good sources, including certain cereals, fruit juice, or milk alternatives. Sunlight is your main source of vitamin D, since your skin produces it when exposed to the sun. However, as you get older, your skin gets less efficient at making it. If you're not out in the sun much or if you cover up your skin, either taking a supplement or increasing food sources of vitamin D may be important. Rich dictary sources include oily fish, eggs, cod liver oil, and foods fortified with vitamin D. A diet rich in calcium and vitamin D is important to prevent the bone loss that can occur during menopause.

2. Maintain a moderate weight

It's common to gain weight during menopause. This can be due to a combination of changing hormones, aging, lifestyle, and genetics. Gaining excess body fat, especially around the waist, increases the risk of developing diseases such as heart disease and diabetes. In addition, body weight may affect menopause symptoms. One study of 17,473 postmenopausal women found that those who lost at least 10 pounds (4.5 kg) of weight or 10% of their body weight over a year were more likely to eliminate hot flashes and night sweats. Achieving and maintaining a healthy weight may help alleviate menopause symptoms and help prevent disease.

3. Eat lots of fruit and vegetables

A diet rich in fruits and vegetables can help prevent a number of menopause symptoms. Fruits and veggies are low in calories and can help you feel full, so they're great for weight loss and weight maintenance. They may also help prevent a number of diseases, including heart disease. This is important, since heart disease risk tends to increase after menopause. This could be due to factors such as age, weight gain, or possibly reduced estrogen levels. Finally, fruits and vegetables may also help prevent bone loss. One observational study of 3,236 women ages 50 to 59 found that diets high in fruit and vegetables may lead to less bone breakdown. A diet rich in fruit and vegetables may help keep bones healthy and can help prevent weight gain and certain diseases.

4. Avoid trigger foods

Certain foods may trigger hot flashes, night sweats, and mood changes. They may be even more likely to be triggers when eaten at night. Common triggers include caffeine, alcohol, and foods that are sugary or spicy. Keep a symptom diary. If you feel that particular foods trigger your menopause symptoms, try to reduce your consumption or avoid them completely. Certain foods and drinks can trigger hot flashes, night sweats, and mood changes. This includes caffeine, alcohol, and sugary or spicy foods.

5. Exercise regularly

There is currently not enough evidence to confirm whether exercise is effective for treating hot flashes and night sweats. However, there is evidence to support other benefits of regular exercise, such as Pilates-based exercise programs. These benefits include improved energy and metabolism, healthier joints and bones, decreased stress, and better sleep. For example, a study in Korea that looked at the effects of a 12-week walking exercise program found that the exercise improved physical and mental health and overall quality of life in a group of 40 menopausal women. Regular exercise is also associated with better overall health and protection against diseases and conditions including cancer, heart disease, stroke, high blood pressure, type 2 diabetes, obesity, and osteoporosis. Menopausal people have a notable increase in heart disease risk; several studies show that regular exercise may help reduce this risk. Regular exercise can help alleviate menopause symptoms such as poor sleep, anxiety, low mood, and fatigue. It can also protect against weight gain and various diseases and conditions.

6. Eat more foods that are high in phytoestrogens

Phytoestrogens are naturally occurring plant compounds that can mimic the effects of estrogen in the body. Therefore, they may help balance hormones. The high intake of phytoestrogens in Asian countries such as Japan is thought to be the reason why menopausal people in these places rarely experience hot flashes.Foods rich in phytoestrogens include:

soybeans and soy products

tofu

tempeh

flaxseeds

linseeds

sesame seeds

beans

However, the phytoestrogen content in foods varies depending on processing methods. One study found that diets high in soy were associated with reduced cholesterol levels, blood pressure, and reduced severity of hot flashes and night sweats among women participants who were starting to enter menopause. However, the debate continues over whether soy products are good or bad for health. Evidence suggests that real food sources of phytoestrogens are better than supplements or processed foods with added soy protein. Foods rich in phytoestrogens may have modest benefits for hot flashes and heart disease risk. However, the evidence is mixed.

7. Drink enough water

During menopause, dryness is often an issue. This is likely caused by the decrease in estrogen levels. Drinking 8 to 12 glasses of water a day can help with these symptoms. Drinking water can also reduce the bloating that can occur with hormonal changes.

In addition, water can help prevent weight gain and aid in weight loss by helping you feel full and increasing metabolism slightly (19Trusted Source, 20Trusted Source).

Drinking 17 ounces (500 ml) of water, 30 minutes before a meal, may lead you to consume 13% fewer calories during the meal. Drinking enough water may help prevent weight gain, aid in weight loss, and reduce symptoms of dryness.

8. Reduce refined sugar and processed foods

A diet high in refined carbs and sugar can cause sharp rises and dips in blood sugar, making you feel tired and irritable. This may worsen the physical and mental symptoms of menopause. In fact, one study found that diets high in refined carbs may increase the risk of depression in postmenopausal women. Diets high in processed foods may also affect bone health, especially if these foods are replacing the nutrients you need from a daily balanced diet. A large observational study found that among women ages 50 to 59, diets high in processed and snack foods were associated with poor bone quality. Diets high in processed foods and refined carbs are associated with a higher risk of depression and worse bone health in postmenopausal people.

9. Don't skip meals

Eating regular meals may be important when you're going through menopause. Irregular eating may make certain symptoms of menopause worse and make weight management more difficult. A yearlong weight management program for postmenopausal women found that skipping meals was associated with 4.3% less weight loss. Irregular eating may cause some symptoms of menopause to worsen. Skipping meals may also hinder weight loss and management during postmenopause.

10. Eat protein-rich foods

Regularly eating protein throughout the day can help prevent the loss of lean muscle mass that occurs with age. One study found that consuming protein throughout the day at each meal may slow down muscle loss due to aging. In addition to helping prevent muscle loss, high protein diets can help with weight loss because they enhance fullness and increase the number of calories burned. Foods rich in protein include meat, fish, eggs, legumes, nuts, and dairy.

11. Take natural supplements

Many people may consider taking natural products and remedies to relieve their menopause symptoms. But the evidence behind many of them is weak.

Your Menopause Meal Plan for Symptom Support

Diet isn't usually the first line of defense for treating menopause symptoms. Still, that doesn't mean that the foods you eat don't play a significant role in how you feel during this phase of life. Crafting your diet with informed choices can help reduce inflammation, balance hormone levels, and even support relief for specific menopause symptoms like hot flashes and mood changes. Plus, planning out your meals offers a comforting sense of self-care when it feels like your hormones are spinning out of control.Here are a host of options for breakfast, lunch, dinner, and snacks for menopause support that are delicious and easy to follow. Let's dig in!

Breakfast

Soy yogurt parfait

For years, rumors have swirled around soy's potentially negative effects on hormones. Don't let the internet chatter fool you. Soy foods are actually a great choice during menopause. "Soy-based foods contain phytoestrogens, which are plant compounds that mimic estrogen in the body," said Julie Pace, RDN, who specializes in functional nutrition for women. Estrogen levels decline during menopause, leading to symptoms like hot flashes and mood changes. "Phytoestrogens can help alleviate these symptoms by providing a mild estrogenic effect," said Pace

Try it

Whip up a soy-based parfait for breakfast by mixing 1 tub soy yogurt, 1/2 cup of berries of your choice, and 2 tablespoons (tbsp) walnut pieces.

Nutty flaxseed and berry smoothie

Ground flaxseeds contain lignans, a type of phytoestrogen, which means they can help turn down the heat of menopause. A 2019 study found that eating these seeds had positive effects on menopause symptoms like hot flashes.

Try it

Reap their benefits at breakfast by blending:

1 tbsp ground flaxseed

1/2 a frozen banana

1 cup milk of your choice

1/2 cup frozen mixed berries

1 tbsp nut butter

Top with a dusting of cinnamon or nutmeg.

Whole wheat avocado toast

Morning decreases in estrogen can raiseTrusted Source your cortisol levels, leaving you feeling anxious first thing. Su-Nui Escobar, DCN, RDN, FAND, of Menopause Better, suggests easing morning nerves by mashing some eggy avocado toast. "This breakfast has both protein and healthy fats, which can decrease morning anxiety," she says.

Try it

Toast your bread to your liking and spread half a ripe avocado over the toast. Then top the whole thing with an over-hard fried egg.

Lunch

Green salad with turmeric-lemon dressing and salmon

Forgetfulness and brain fog can be common in menopause as hormones ebb and flow. A dose of curcumin, the active ingredient in turmeric, may help. "Curcumin may help improve memory by lowering brain inflammation," said Escobar. Add the inflammation-fighting benefits of curcumin to a fresh green salad topped with baked salmon. Remember to add black pepper to reap the benefits of curcumin.

Try it

Add four salmon filets to a baking dish. In a small bowl, mix 1 tbsp lemon juice, 2 teaspoons (tsp) garlic, and salt and pepper to taste. Spoon over the salmon and bake for 15 minutes at 400°F. As a side, grab a bag of mixed salad greens from the store. Escobar recommends the following lemon-turmeric dressing for drizzling:

1/4 cup olive oil

2 tbsp lemon juice

1/2 tsp ground turmeric

1/2 tsp ground ginger

1/2 tbsp honey

1/2 tbsp finely chopped shallot

1 tsp or more black pepper

salt, to taste

Southwestern baked sweet potato

A baked sweet potato not only packs well for an on-the-go lunch — it's got plenty of fiber to fight menopause constipation. A sprinkle of pumpkin seeds finishes things off with vitamin E and magnesium. "Vitamin E may help to reduce hot flashes and support skin health during menopause," said Pace. "Magnesium can help with muscle relaxation, improve sleep, and reduce anxiety."

Try it

Bake a sweet potato until tender. An hour at 425°F is usually sufficient. Once it's cooled, top with rinsed, drained black beans (more fiber!), salsa, and avocado slices. Sprinkle pumpkin seeds on top to your liking.

Vegan sushi bowl

Believe it or not, sushi doesn't have to contain fish! Try a nutrient-rich, menopause-supporting sushi bowl that's totally plant-based. You can create a hormone-friendly lunch with a few simple ingredients. The estrogenic effects of edamame and sesame seeds may help tame hot flashes, while the quinoa and vegetables round out the dish's fiber content.

Try it

Begin with a bed of cooked quinoa, then add steamed edamame, avocado slices, sesame seeds, cucumber, and any other vegetables you favor. A topping of crispy fried onions or a cashew-based cream sauce to complete the vegan picture.

Dinner

Beef meatballs with flaxseed

If your perimenopause journey has you menstruating for lengthy stretches, you may be at risk of iron-deficiency anemia. Adding iron-rich beef to your diet can help restore your energy levels. (And if you add flaxseeds to the mix, you'll amp up phytoestrogens for even more menopause support.) These hidden-flaxseed meatballs are a winning combination that serves four.

Try it

Mix the following in a large bowl:

1 lb ground beef

1 egg white

1/3 cup ground flaxseed

3 tbsp parmesan cheese

1 tbsp olive oil

1 tsp minced garlic

1/2 tsp salt

1/4 tsp black pepper

1/2 tsp dried oregano

1 tsp dried basil

Form into 1-inch balls and bake on a greased baking sheet in a 350°F oven for 30 minutes or until meatballs reach an internal temperature of 145°F.

Tofu vegetable stirfry

Need more evidence that soy is a ticket to menopausal health? A 2021 study revealed that a plant-based diet rich in soy reduced moderate-to-severe hot flashes by 84%. Over the course of the 12-week study, nearly 60% of participants eliminated moderate-to-severe hot flashes. Stick with soy by enjoying a simple, single-serving tofu vegetable stirfry for dinner.

Try it

Sauté 3 oz cubed extra-firm tofu in 1/2 tbsp vegetable oil until browned, then add veggies of your choice (bell peppers, broccoli, onions, or cauliflower, to name a few). Splash on your favorite store-bought or homemade stirfry marinade and serve over 1 cup of cooked brown rice.

Salmon, beans, and greens

You've probably heard about the inflammation-fighting benefits of omega-3 fatty acids. Their potential for busting inflammation on a systemic level may help alleviate some of the symptoms of menopause. "Menopause itself is an inflammatory process, and the benefits of omega-3 fatty acids from fish can help reduce inflammation," said Escobar.

Try it

Make the salmon:

Drizzle a salmon filet with olive oil and lemon juice and sprinkle with salt, pepper, and garlic powder. Bake at

425°F for about 15 minutes or until the fish flakes easily. Make the side:

Heat 1/2 tbsp olive oil in a large skillet over medium heat.

Add 2 cloves minced garlic and sauté until fragrant.

Add 2 cups chopped kale and 1/2 cup rinsed, drained white beans.

Cook until the beans are heated through and the kale has wilted.

Season with salt and pepper to taste, then serve salmon atop kale and beans.

Snacks and desserts

Curry turmeric popcorn

Turmeric is more versatile than you might think. How about trying its anti-inflammatory zing on popcorn?

Try it

For a savory snack, pop a bag of plain microwave popcorn and transfer to a large bowl. In a small bowl, stir together:

2 tbsp olive oil

1 tsp curry powder

1/2 tsp turmeric

1/2 tsp salt

1/2 tsp pepper

1/8 tsp cayenne powder

Drizzle the oil mixture over the popcorn, stirring well to coat.

Chia seed pudding

Chia seeds earn their "superfood" title by packing an abundance of nutrients into an itty-bitty package. It just so happens that many of these nutrients may help relieve menopause symptoms. Chia seedsTrusted Source are rich in omega-3 fats and contain magnesium, calcium, phosphorus, and potassium, all of which support a smooth menopausal transition.

At snack time or dessert, amp up your nutrition with an easy chia seed pudding.

Try it

Place 2 tbsp chia seeds, 1/2 cup almond milk, and 1 tsp maple syrup to a Mason jar.

Mix well, cover, and refrigerate for at least 2 hours.

Finish it off with your favorite berries, peach slices, chocolate chips, or nuts.

Steamed edamame

Morning, noon, or night, edamame is an excellent anytime snack for menopause! Its phytoestrogens can prevent or reduce the severity of hot flashes, while its fiber content (8 grams per cupTrusted Source) improves the potential digestive troubles of menopause.

Try it

Snag a microwaveable frozen bag of edamame and steam according to package directions, or pick up a ready-to-eat vacuum-sealed pack.

Maca peanut butter energy balls

Maca root is a Peruvian adaptogen that's been studied for its ability to calm multiple menopause symptoms. A 2022 systematic review concluded that maca root may have significant effects on menopause-related problems, including memory impairment, depression, and bone structure changes. If you're new to using maca root in recipes, start small with these simple energy balls.

Try it

In the bowl of a food processor, combine 1 cup pitted Medjool dates, 1 cup walnuts, and 1/2 cup peanut butter. Process until the nuts are finely chopped.

Add 3 tbsp maca powder, 3/4 cup rolled oats, and 2 tbsp water. Process until smooth and malleable.

Form into 1-inch balls and store in the refrigerator.

Dark chocolate-covered strawberries

It's not uncommon to crave sweets when your hormones are all over the map. Satisfy a sweet tooth with dark chocolate-covered strawberries. The antioxidants in chocolate have been associatedTrusted Source with improved cognition and reduced fatigue.

Try it

Dip washed, dried whole strawberries into your favorite melted chocolate chips. Pace recommends a 70% or higher cacao level for mood enhancement. Let the chocolate harden before eating — if you can wait that long!

No one ever said going through menopause was fun, but taking charge of your diet can provide a sense of empowerment for your hormone health. A few informed food choices can see you through the journey with better nutrition, fewer physical symptoms, and a sunnier outlook.

CONCLUSION

Mostwomenbeginmenopausebetweentheagesof45and55.Th eaverageageformenopauseonsetintheUnitedStatesis51years old.Earlymenopauseusuallyreferstoonsetbeforeage45.Prema turemenopauseorprematureovarianinsufficiencyoccursbefor eage40..Menopauseoccurswhenyourovariesstopproducinge ggs,resultinginlowestrogenlevels.Estrogenisthehormonethat controlsthereproductivecycle.Someoneisinmenopausewhent heyhaven'thadaperiodformorethan12months.Butassociateds ymptoms,suchashotflashes,startlongbeforemenopausedurin gaphasecalledperimenopause.

www.ingramcontent.com/pod-product-compliance
Lightning Source LLC
Chambersburg PA
CBHW061013260726
48661CB00005B/2178